Yoni Steaming With CBD for Beginners

Explore the ancient practice of integrating CBD for transforming feminine well-being.

Title:
Yoni Steaming With CBD for Beginners

Subtitle

Explore the ancient practice of integrating CBD for transforming feminine well-being.

Copyright © 2023 by (Guillermo Bode MD)

Printed in the United States of America.

ISBN: 9798872474982

TABLE OF CONTENT

INTRODUCTION

Cannabidiol Yoni Steaming is a holistic approach to feminine wellness that blends the ancient technique of Yoni Steaming with the therapeutic advantages of cannabidiol. We would like to use this opportunity to welcome you to the interesting world of that practice (CBD). Beginning with the fundamental ideas that will serve as the basis for our investigation, this introductory chapter will go into those ideas.

Understanding Yoni Steaming

The practice of Yoni Steaming, which is sometimes referred to as vaginal steaming or V-steam, is an age-old method that has been utilized in a variety of civilizations for hundreds of years. In Sanskrit, the term "Yoni" refers to the female genitalia, but it is also frequently used to refer to the reproductive system as a whole. When performing Yoni Steaming, the practitioner sits over a pot of herbal steam to allow the warmth and moisture to permeate the vaginal tissues that are located on the outside. It is claimed that the technique originated in several different cultures, including traditional Chinese medicine and Mayan traditions. In these societies, it was utilized to improve the reproductive health of women, maintain hormonal balance, and treat a variety of gynecological disorders.

It is necessary to have an understanding of the philosophy that Yoni Steaming is based on to fully comprehend the practice. This philosophy is based on the concept that the female reproductive system is a sacred space that deserves to be cared for and attended to. Yoni Steaming is considered to be a therapeutic and ceremonial practice that helps women feel more connected to their bodies, fosters feelings of self-love, and enhances their general well-being. Women have experienced a variety of benefits as a result of participating in this ancient practice, including a reduction in the severity of menstrual cramps and an increase

in feelings of sensuality.

The Integration of CBD in Yoni Steaming

Yoni Steaming has been given a modern makeover with the use of CBD, which combines traditional wisdom with modern holistic wellness. Cannabidiol, also known as CBD, is a non-psychoactive substance with several medicinal uses that are present in cannabis plants. To maximize the potential health advantages of Yoni Steaming, CBD can be integrated by adding CBD-rich herbs or infusing the herbal steam with CBD oil.

Yoni steaming benefits from the special qualities that CBD offers, such as its anti-inflammatory, analgesic, and calming effects. These qualities can enhance the conventional advantages of yoni steaming, providing a more all-encompassing strategy for the well-being of women. The endocannabinoid system, which is essential for controlling some physiological functions like mood, pain perception, and inflammation, is influenced by interactions between the cannabinoids in CBD. People want to utilize these therapeutic effects for a more profound and comprehensive experience by adding CBD to Yoni steaming.

Benefits of CBD Yoni Steaming

A vast array of physical, mental, and spiritual facets of women's health are improved by CBD yoni steaming. The following benefits are anecdotally recorded, however, it's important to note that individual experiences may differ as we examine this chapter:

Pain Reduction and Decreased Soreness: Thanks to its analgesic qualities, CBD may help reduce soreness during Yoni Steaming sessions. Women have reported less pelvic pain, less menstrual cramps, and relief from discomfort related to a variety of gynecological conditions.

Hormonal Balance: Yoni steaming and CBD is thought to help with hormonal balance. People may benefit from fewer PMS symptoms, more regular menstrual cycles, and enhanced hormonal balance by treating any possible reproductive system imbalances.

Improved Stress Reduction and Relaxation: CBD is well known for its anxiolytic (stress-relieving) qualities. When included in Yoni Steaming, CBD may help practitioners feel more at ease, reduce stress, and have a higher level of emotional well-being both during and after the practice.

Enhanced Sensuality and Connection to Body: Yoni steaming, in conjunction with the use of CBD, is frequently linked to heightened sensuality and a closer bond with one's body. This stronger bond could result in better sex, more self-assurance, and a better perception of one's body in general.

Support for Reproductive Health: CBD may provide further support for the reproductive system, which has historically been associated with yoni steaming. A few women report feeling better overall about their reproductive health, as well as improvements in their ability to conceive and produce more cervical mucus.

CHAPTER 1: THE BASICS OF YONI STEAMING

An ancient technique that has its origins in a wide variety of cultures all over the world, Yoni Steaming is a strategy that takes a holistic approach to the reproductive health and well-being of women. The purpose of this chapter is to investigate the fundamental components of Yoni Steaming, including its definition, the historical context in which it has been practiced, and the mechanics that govern how this centuries-old custom operates.

What is Yoni Steaming?

The technique known as Yoni Steaming is based on the utilization of herbal steam to nourish and revitalize the pelvic region. This technique encompasses the exterior tissues of the vagina as well as the areas surrounding it. The term "Yoni" comes from the Sanskrit language and refers to the female reproductive organs. Furthermore, Yoni Steaming is frequently referred to as vaginal steaming or V-steam.

Within the context of the practice, a lady is generally seen seated or crouching over a pot of steam that contains herbal infusions. A mixture of particular herbs is simmered in water, which causes the herbs' beneficial compounds to be released, which results in the production of steam. These medicinal herbs have been selected with great care due to the numerous therapeutic properties that they possess, which may include anti-inflammatory, antibacterial, and toning effects.

It is believed that the warmth and moisture that the steam provides might help to improve circulation, relax the muscles in the pelvic region, and support the natural cleansing processes that occur within the body. Yoni Steaming is frequently regarded as a ritualistic exercise that promotes self-care and helps to cultivate a connection between a woman and her body.

Historical Context and Cultural Practices

Yoni steaming has its origins in many cultures and traditions, where it was seen as a healing and spiritual practice for women's reproductive health. Let's examine a few of the historical and cultural settings that have influenced Yoni Steaming's development:

Traditional Chinese Medicine (TCM): For millennia, Yoni Steaming, sometimes referred to as "chai-yok," has been used in TCM. It is thought to enhance general reproductive health, control menstrual cycles, and increase blood circulation. Based on each person's demands and concerns, different herbal mixtures are used.

Mayan Tradition: As a means of purification and spiritual connection, the ancient Mayans engaged in a sort of yoni steaming. Utilizing herbal steam to balance reproductive energy and cleanse the uterus was the procedure known as "bajo."

African and Native American customs: Steam baths have long been associated with health benefits for women in several African and Native American civilizations. Herbs from the area were added to the steam to treat specific gynecological problems and enhance general health.

Korean Tradition: In Korea, a comparable custom called "chai-yok" entails consuming a hot pot of therapeutic herbs. This custom, which has been handed down through the years, is frequently seen as a postpartum healing technique.

The variety of these cultural customs emphasizes how widespread it is to see the female reproductive system as a sacred component of women's health and to acknowledge and take care of it.

How Yoni Steaming Works

Yoni Steaming works by combining the infusion of herbs with steam and the body's natural healing processes. This is an explanation of Yoni Steaming's operation:

Herbal Selection: Certain plants are picked out specifically because of their medicinal qualities. Herbs including calendula, mugwort, rosemary, chamomile, and basil are often used. The ability of these herbs to tonify, cleanse, and calm the reproductive tissues is generally the deciding factor in their selection.

Herbal Steam Production: The chosen herbs are infused with hot water to produce a steam that has the medicinal qualities of the plants. The steam is kept at a moderate temperature so that it is comforting and warm rather than scorching.

Sitting Over the Steam: The woman takes a seat over the herbal steam pot and covers her lower body with a cloth or blanket to keep the steam contained. The steam rises and covers the perineum and external genitalia.

Purifying and Nourishing: It is thought that the steam's warmth will improve blood flow, soothe tense muscles, and encourage the production of vaginal secretions. It is believed that this procedure supports general reproductive health, facilitates detoxification, and cleanses the reproductive organs.

Beyond the physical, yoni steaming frequently entails a spiritual and emotional connection as well as an intention. During this period, women can make plans, engage in mindfulness exercises, and develop a closer relationship with their bodies.

Remember that yoni steaming is a complementary therapy and should never be used in place of medical attention. Even though many women have had good results with yoni steaming, it's still essential for people to speak with medical specialists, particularly if they have any underlying health issues or concerns.

CHAPTER 2: CBD AND ITS THERAPEUTIC PROPERTIES

Cannabidiol, also known as CBD, has garnered a lot of attention in recent years when it comes to the possible therapeutic characteristics it possesses. The purpose of this chapter is to provide a full overview of cannabidiol (CBD), including an examination of its history, the health benefits it offers, and the unique implications it has for the health of women.

Introduction to CBD (Cannabidiol)

The cannabis plant contains approximately 100 different types of cannabinoids, of which CBD is one. Tetrahydrocannabinol (THC), the more well-known counterpart of CBD, is not psychoactive, meaning it does not result in a "high" feeling. Both hemp and marijuana plants can be used to make CBD, although hemp is the preferred source because of its lower THC level.

Interaction with the Endocannabinoid System (ECS): The endocannabinoid system is a sophisticated cell-signaling system found in the human body that regulates several bodily processes, including mood, appetite, sleep patterns, and immune response. Through its effects on receptors like CB1 and CB2, CBD interacts with the endocannabinoid system to preserve homeostasis and enhance general well-being.

CBD can be found in many different forms, such as oils, tinctures, capsules, edibles, topicals, and more. People can select the approach that best meets their needs and tastes from among the several forms, each of which has advantages and things to keep in mind.

Legal Aspects: CBD has different legal statuses around the world. Legal in many states as long as the THC content is less than 0.3 percent, CBD made from hemp is. On the other hand, people must understand and abide by the laws in their particular area.

Gaining an understanding of the fundamentals of CBD is essential before delving into its possible health advantages and applications in integrative wellness regimens.

Health Benefits of CBD

Pain Relief and Anti-Inflammatory Effects: The ability of CBD to lessen pain and inflammation is one of its most well-known advantages. CBD is a popular option for those with chronic pain disorders since studies have shown that it may interact with the immune system and brain receptors to reduce pain and inflammation.

Anxiety and Stress Reduction: CBD has shown anxiolytic (anxiety-reducing) qualities, which suggests that it might be a good choice for people with anxiety problems. It modifies mood and stress reactions via interacting with brain receptors, including serotonin receptors.

Better Sleep: By addressing issues like anxiety and pain that lead to sleep disturbances, CBD has demonstrated the potential to support better sleep. CBD may assist in controlling sleep cycles and enhancing the general quality of sleep by interacting with the endocannabinoid system.

Neuroprotective Properties: Studies indicate that CBD may help people with neurodegenerative diseases by having neuroprotective qualities. These results have raised interest in CBD as a possible therapeutic agent for diseases like multiple sclerosis and Alzheimer's disease, while additional research is required.

Anti-Seizure Effects: Epidiolex, a CBD-based medicine, was approved by the U.S. Food and Drug Administration (FDA) for the treatment of epilepsy after CBD was shown to be able to lessen the frequency and severity of seizures in certain forms of epilepsy.

Anti-Nausea and Appetite Stimulation: CBD may be able to reduce nausea and increase appetite, especially in patients receiving chemotherapy or suffering from illnesses that impair appetite.

Cardiovascular Health: Research indicates that CBD may reduce blood pressure and have other positive effects on the cardiovascular system.

The total cardioprotective benefits of CBD are influenced by these possible effects on the cardiovascular system.

A more comprehensive understanding of these health advantages offers insight into the various ways that CBD can enhance general well-being. It's important to understand the particular ways that CBD interacts with the female body before delving into the consequences for women's health.

CBD and Women's Health

Menstrual Pain and Discomfort: During their menstrual cycles, many women suffer from menstrual cramps and pain. Because of its anti-inflammatory and analgesic qualities, CBD may provide relief by lowering menstrual pain and inflammation.

Hormonal Balance: The endocannabinoid system, which is essential for controlling hormones, is impacted by CBD. Based on this interaction, it appears that CBD may help maintain hormonal balance. This is especially important for women going through menopause, pregnancy, and other life transitions.

Menopause symptoms include mood swings, hot flashes, and sleep disruptions brought on by the hormonal changes that accompany menopause. Because CBD can improve sleep, lower anxiety, and regulate mood, it may help women going through menopause.

Reproductive Health: The possible effects of CBD on reproductive health have been investigated. Although studies are still being conducted, some indicate that CBD may affect fertility via controlling parameters related to reproductive health and interacting with the endocannabinoid system.

Stress Management and Mental Health Issues: Women frequently balance a variety of tasks and obligations, which increases their risk of developing stress-related mental health issues. The anxiolytic qualities of CBD may be especially advantageous for stress reduction and promoting mental health in general.

Skin Health: The antioxidant and anti-inflammatory qualities of CBD also benefit skin health. Women looking to treat conditions including inflammation, acne, and aging symptoms may want to look at skincare products with added CBD.

It is noteworthy to acknowledge that although CBD exhibits the potential to address multiple facets of women's health, subjective reactions may differ. As with any supplement or wellness regimen, speaking with medical specialists is advised, particularly for women who are expecting or nursing as well as those who have underlying medical issues.

CHAPTER 3: GETTING STARTED WITH CBD YONI STEAMING

The process of CBD Yoni Steaming requires careful consideration of needed tools, the selection of acceptable CBD products, and the observance of safety precautions before beginning the voyage. In this chapter, you will find a thorough guide that will assist you in beginning this holistic wellness practice.

Essential Tools and Supplies

To guarantee a comfortable and successful experience, it's imperative to obtain the necessary equipment and supplies before beginning CBD yo-steaming. This is a summary of what you will require:

Yoni Steam Herbs: The key to a successful yoni steaming session is choosing the appropriate herbs. Herbs including mugwort, rosemary, chamomile, calendula, and basil are frequently used in yoni steaming. These plants have a variety of medicinal qualities, including actions that include calming, purifying, and toning. To maximize the potential advantages of CBD Yoni Steaming, think about adding herbs high in CBD or herbal combinations infused with CBD.

Steamer or Yoni Steam Seat: You'll need a special steamer or Yoni steam seat to speed up the steaming procedure. These are made to make it possible to sit comfortably over a steaming pot of herbs. While some solutions are easy to use and portable, others are made to be positioned over toilets. Select a seat or steamer based on your needs and preferences.

Big Pot or Steaming Equipment: To make herbal steam in a more do-it-yourself manner, use a big pot or steaming device. Make sure it is stable and resistant to heat. To keep the steam contained and avoid losing too much heat, you'll need a cover.

Blanket or Shawl: During the steaming process, a blanket or shawl is necessary to create a warm and enclosed area. This improves the practice's efficacy by keeping the steam contained and the temperature stable.

Select a Cozy Chair or Cushion: The Yoni steam seat should be positioned on a cozy chair or cushion. By doing this, you may be confident that you'll be able to have a calm and relaxed posture the entire session.

Huge Robe or Towel: It's useful to have a big robe or towel close by so you can cover up before, during, and after the session. This enhances coziness and aids in maintaining warmth.

CBD-infused Oil or Salve (Optional): Although the herbs in the steam offer a holistic experience, some people want to boost the CBD component by applying an oil or salve rich with CBD. For extra therapeutic results, this can be applied externally to the pelvic area or perineum.

Gathering these necessary equipment and materials will help you set up a comfortable space for your CBD Yoni Steaming session.

Choosing the Right CBD Products

A crucial part of adding CBD to your Yoni Steaming regimen is choosing the appropriate CBD products. When selecting CBD products for this practice, keep the following points in mind:

CBD quality: Give top priority to premium CBD products sourced from reliable vendors. Seek for goods that have undergone independent testing to ensure their efficacy and purity. This guarantees that the CBD source you're using is trustworthy and secure.

CBD Concentration: Take into account the product's CBD concentration. Because concentrations can differ, pick a product based on your tastes and intended outcomes. Novices might begin with lower concentrations and work their way up as needed.

Recognize the distinctions between full-spectrum, broad-spectrum, and isolate CBD products. Full-spectrum products have a small quantity of THC among other cannabinoids (within legal limits). While CBD isolate is pure CBD, broad-spectrum products contain several cannabinoids without THC. Full-spectrum products are frequently linked to the entourage effect, in which cannabinoids collaborate harmoniously.

Method of Consumption: There are several ways to consume CBD, such as oils, tinctures, capsules, and topicals. Use CBD tincture or oil for yoni steaming; these can be readily incorporated into the herbal steam. Alternatively, if you would rather apply it externally, the perineum can be treated with an oil or salve loaded with CBD.

Organic and Natural Components: Make sure that the goods infused with CBD are created using organic and natural ingredients if you decide to purchase them. This is consistent with Yoni Steaming's natural and comprehensive approach.

Scent and Additional Ingredients: For aroma and extra medicinal effects, certain CBD products may contain additional botanicals or essential oils. Think about your individual preferences and any sensitivity you might have to particular chemicals or smells.

Dosage & Customization: The appropriate dosage of CBD varies from person to person, so it's important to determine what works best for you. Take less at first, and if necessary, increase it gradually. Customization is essential, so observe how your body reacts and make the necessary adjustments.

Yoni Steaming has several therapeutic effects that can be further enhanced by selecting premium CBD products that suit your needs and preferences.

Safety Precautions

As with any wellness practice, CBD Yoni Steaming should always be done with utmost safety. The following are crucial safety measures to think about:

Consultation with Healthcare Professionals: See your doctor before starting a CBD Yoni Steaming regimen, particularly if you have any underlying medical concerns or are nursing a baby. Although many women find yoni steaming to be helpful, each person's health situation is different.

Allergies and Sensitivities: Be aware of any dietary restrictions or any allergies you may have to herbs or CBD products. Choose carefully which herbs and CBD products suit your sensitivities if you have known allergies, or speak with a herbalist or healthcare professional.

Temperature Moderation: Make sure the herbal steam is heated to a safe and comfortable level. To prevent pain or burns, the steam should be warm rather than hot. Throughout the practice, pay attention to your body's cues and take breaks as needed.

Avoiding Irritants: Steer clear of douches, abrasive soaps, and other potentially irritating items both before and after yoni steaming.

Permit the vaginal environment to remain in its natural balance.

Maintain Good Hygiene: Before and after the session, wash your hands to uphold good hygiene. Maintain the cleanliness and hygienic storage of the equipment and materials used for yoni steaming.

Moderation and Frequency: It is typically advised to use yoni steaming, including CBD yoni steaming, in moderation. The vaginal microbiome's natural balance may be upset by excessive steaming. If you'd like, start with shorter sessions and progressively extend them.

Effects Monitoring: Observe your body's reaction to CBD Yoni Steaming. Stop the practice and seek medical advice if you feel any discomfort, irritability, or strange symptoms.

Privacy and Comfort: For your Yoni Steaming sessions, pick a quiet, cozy area. Establish a space where you may unwind and devote yourself to the exercise without any distractions.

You can make thoughtful and responsible use of the advantages of CBD Yoni Steaming by putting safety first and adhering to these guidelines.

CHAPTER 4: DIY CBD YONI STEAMING RECIPES

Unlocking the full potential of CBD Yoni Steaming requires the creation of individualized herbal blends that are tailored to the specific requirements of each individual. This chapter will walk you through the process of creating CBD-infused herbal mixes, adjusting recipes to meet your unique needs, and providing advice on how to have a session that is both pleasant and productive.

Creating CBD-infused Herbal Blends

A DIY CBD Yoni Steaming session starts with carefully choosing herbs, especially ones high in CBD, to make a blend that specifically targets your wellness objectives. This is a detailed tutorial on making herbal mixtures with CBD for Yoni Steaming:

Select a Base Herb: As the base of your blend, start with this herb. Because of its cleaning and toning qualities, mugwort is a popular option. Calendula, chamomile, rosemary, and lavender are further choices. Think about each herb's medicinal qualities and how they fit with your objectives.

Add Herbs High in CBD: To increase the blend's potential benefits, add herbs rich in CBD. You can add hemp leaves and flowers, which are high in CBD, to the mixture. You can also experiment with other herbs like black pepper and catnip that are recognized for having high cannabinoid content.

Choose Extra Herbs for Particular Advantages: Customize your mixture by including herbs that deal with particular issues. Consider adding chamomile or lavender for relaxation. Try dong quai or red clover for hormonal balance. Examine the characteristics of several herbs to develop a concoction that complements your health objectives.

Try experimenting with aromatics: these herbs enhance all the senses in addition to providing smell. To make the steam smell even better, try adding a tiny bit of aromatic herbs like yarrow, jasmine, or rose petals.

Balance the Blend: By adding herbs in the right amounts, you may create a harmonic blend. Though there are no hard and fast guidelines, take into account the strength of each herb and try to create a well-balanced combination that appeals to your senses.

Infuse with CBD Oil: You can incorporate CBD oil into your herbal combination to give it an added boost. Make sure the CBD oil has the appropriate concentration and is of excellent quality. Depending on your tastes, start with a few drops and work your way up.

Store in a Cold, Dark Area: To maintain the freshness and potency of the herbs, store your CBD-infused herbal blend in a cool, dark place after you've produced it. Try storing the blend in an airtight container to keep moisture from damaging it.

By experimenting with various herbs and CBD dosages, you can make a customized combination that supports your wellness goals.

Tailoring Recipes to Individual Needs

The versatility of DIY CBD Yoni Steaming recipes makes them incredibly attractive. Take into account the following while personalizing your recipes:

Period: Adjust the herbal blend to suit your menstrual cycle. For instance, in the follicular phase, use toning herbs like mugwort, and in the luteal phase, use relaxing herbs like chamomile.

Particular Health Objectives: Determine your unique health objectives and select herbs that support them. Use relaxing herbs, such as lavender, if your goal is stress relief. Look into herbs that are recognized to have adaptogenic qualities for hormonal balance.

Sensory Preferences: Take them into account when choosing herbs. Add rose petals or jasmine if you like floral scents. Try using herbs like sage or rosemary for a more earthy scent. A combination that appeals to your senses improves the whole experience.

Frequency and Length: Adapt the length and frequency of your Yoni Steaming sessions to your requirements and comfort zone. While some people want longer sessions less frequently, others might choose shorter sessions more regularly. Take note of your body's cues and make the necessary adjustments.

Intuitive Herbal Selection: When choosing herbs, follow your instincts. If there is a particular herb that speaks to you or has good connotations, think about adding it to your blend. The activity of choosing herbs gains a personal and spiritual dimension from its intuitive component.

Seasonal Variations: Use herbs that are in season to create interesting seasonal concoctions. This adds variation to your Yoni Steaming regimen and is in line with the natural cycles.

Customizing recipes to meet your specific needs guarantees that your CBD Yoni Steaming experience will suit your particular tastes and wellness goals in addition to being effective.

Tips for a Relaxing and Effective Session

More is involved in achieving a calming and successful CBD Yoni Steaming experience than just the herbal blend. The following advice will improve your overall experience:

Establish a Sacred Location: Make a cozy and sacred space to set the mood for your Yoni Steaming session. Play calming music, turn up soft lighting, and include accessories that promote mindfulness and relaxation.

Approach your Yoni Steaming session with mindfulness by practicing mindfulness. Let go of outside stresses, concentrate on your breathing, and stay in the present. A deeper experience is facilitated and the mind-body connection is strengthened by mindfulness.

Keep Yourself Hydrated: Both before and after Yoni Steaming, you should be hydrated. By staying hydrated throughout the session, drinking water supports the body's natural detoxifying processes.

Warm Up Gradually: Give the steam time to gradually warm up before beginning a Yoni Steaming session. This keeps you from feeling uncomfortable and lets your body adjust to the increasing heat.

Listen to Your Body: During the session, be aware of the cues your body is sending you. Take breaks as needed if the steam feels too hot or if you are uncomfortable. Your encounter will be safe and enjoyable if you pay attention to your body.

Include Breathwork: Throughout your Yoni Steaming session, focus on taking deep, deliberate breaths. This increases pelvic tissue oxygenation while also encouraging relaxation.

Post-Session Self-Care: Take care of yourself after the session. Do some light stretching, have a warm bath, or partake in other relaxing activities. This increases the advantages of Yoni Steaming.

Writing and Introspection: After every session, think about writing in your journal about your thoughts and experiences. You can monitor changes, identify trends, and strengthen your relationship with Yoni Steaming's holistic elements by engaging in this activity.

Maintaining consistency is essential to reaping the full benefits of CBD yoni steaming, even though you might not see improvements right away after only one session. As you incorporate it into your self-care regimen, see the cumulative impacts.

These pointers can help you design a comprehensive and customized CBD Yoni Steaming experience that supports your wellness objectives and improves your general

sense of well-being.

CHAPTER 5: UNDERSTANDING YOUR BODY

For those who are interested in CBD Yoni Steaming and holistic feminine well-being, it is of the utmost importance to get a profound understanding of their bodies. This chapter discusses the significance of paying attention to the signals that your body sends you, being aware of your menstrual cycle, and engaging in the practice of Yoni Mapping to provide individualized treatment.

Listening to Your Body's Signals

One of the fundamental practices of holistic well-being, which includes CBD Yoni Steaming, is listening to your body. Here's why it matters and some tips for learning to read your body's signals:

Body Awareness: Being aware of how your body expresses its wants and reactions is the first step toward developing body awareness. This encompasses feelings, energies, and bodily experiences. Developing body awareness improves your capacity to make decisions that promote your well-being.

Recognizing Comfort and Discomfort: Pay attention to any feelings of comfort or discomfort that arise during CBD Yoni Steaming. It's critical to pay attention to any symptoms of discomfort, such as extreme heat or inflammation, and modify the session as necessary. On the other hand, warmth and relaxation are signs that the practice is in good alignment with your body.

Mind-Body Connection: A key component of holistic well-being is the mind-body connection. Take part in mindfulness exercises to strengthen the bond between your mind and body, such as meditation and deep breathing.

This relationship improves your capacity to comprehend and react to bodily cues.

Intuitive Decision-Making: When making choices that will affect your health, follow your gut. Often, your body gives you instinctive cues about what feels good or incorrect for you. This is true for many facets of self-care and lifestyle decisions, not only CBD yoni steaming.

Emotional Awareness: Understanding your emotions is essential to knowing your body. Observe the effects that various activities, such as CBD Yoni Steaming, have on your mental health. Recognize and accept any feelings of relaxation or increased sensuality you may be experiencing as a natural component of the whole.

Regularly evaluate your experiences with CBD yoni steaming and other health-related activities. To record your feelings, experiences, and any changes you notice over time, keep a diary. By reflecting regularly, you can spot trends and modify your self-care regimen wisely.

Actively attending to your body's cues helps you develop a closer relationship with yourself and makes holistic wellness more individualized and successful.

Menstrual Cycle Awareness

One important component of feminine well-being is being aware of your menstrual cycle. Tracking your cycle's phases and appreciating the special requirements and advantages of each phase is part of developing menstrual cycle awareness. Menstrual cycle awareness can improve your CBD Yoni Steaming routine in the following ways:

Menstruation, the follicular phase, ovulation, and the luteal phase are the four phases that make up the menstrual cycle. Hormonal variations and unique physiological alterations are characteristics of each phase.

Days 1–14 of the Follicular Phase: Estrogen levels increase throughout this phase, which starts when menstruation starts. This stage is linked to more vitality, inventiveness, and a feeling of rejuvenation. Use toning herbs, such as mugwort, to support a sense of rejuvenation when doing CBD yoni steaming.

Day 14 or thereabouts is considered ovulation. During ovulation, an egg is released from the ovary. A rise in energy and fertility are the hallmarks of this phase. If your focus is on sexuality or conception, now would be a good time to try CBD yoni steaming with herbs that promote relaxation.

Days 15–28 are known as the luteal phase. This stage comes after ovulation and is characterized by elevated progesterone levels. This stage is linked to emotional reflection and getting ready for a possible pregnancy. Herbs like lavender or chamomile that promote emotional well-being are good choices for CBD yoni steaming.

Menstruation (Days 1-7): The uterine lining sheds during menstruation, which signifies the end of the cycle. This stage is frequently used for self-care and relaxation. Yoni CBD Herbs that are calming and toning might be the focus of steaming during menstruation to provide comfort and relaxation.

Personalized Care: By being aware of your menstrual cycle, you can tailor your CBD Yoni Steaming routine to meet the unique requirements of each stage. Adjust the herbal mix, length of session, and frequency to suit your menstrual cycle's energy and needs.

Monitoring Monthly Symptoms: Keep a check on symptoms including mood swings, fluctuating energy levels, and physical discomfort by using menstrual cycle tracking apps or notebooks. You can use this information to anticipate and take care of particular demands at different stages of your cycle.

Menstrual cycle knowledge can help you better match your CBD Yoni Steaming practice with your body's natural rhythm, which will make the experience more peaceful and supportive.

Yoni Mapping for Personalized Care

Yoni mapping is an individual investigation of your anatomy and body's distinct reactions. This procedure helps to create a CBD yoni steaming method that is more customized and unique. To use Yoni Mapping for individualized care, follow these steps:

Recognizing Your Anatomy: Invest some time in learning about the structure of your own Yoni (vagina) and surrounding tissues. This entails learning about the interior and external anatomy of the vaginal canal, clitoris, and labia. Being aware of your anatomy can help you feel confident and empowered.

Investigation of Sensations: To comprehend the distinct feelings and reactions of your Yoni, engage in self-examination. This can be self-massaging, using a gentle touch, or just observing how different parts of your Yoni react to stimuli. Yoni mapping promotes a healthy, mutually agreeable relationship with your own body.

Identification of Sensitivities: You can use Yoni mapping to pinpoint sensitive areas or particular preferences. When using CBD yoni steaming, this knowledge is helpful since it lets you customize the technique to your preferences and degree of comfort.

Integration of CBD-infused Products: To ensure compatibility with your skin, conduct a patch test on a small area before using any CBD-infused oils, salves, or creams during Yoni Mapping. To accommodate your preferences and sensitivity, take into account the CBD concentration and any extra substances.

Embracing Personal Preferences: Yoni mapping gives you the chance to accept your boundaries and preferences. While some people might prefer a milder approach, others might prefer a more direct stimulus. You can provide a secure and encouraging environment for self-care behaviors by acknowledging and respecting your personal preferences.

Exploration with Mindfulness: When doing Yoni mapping, keep your attention in the here and now and develop a healthy relationship with your body. Your capacity to pay attention to and act on your body's cues improves with mindful investigation.

Ritual Integration: Take into Account Including Rituals in Your Yoni Mapping Practice. Creating a sacred area, lighting candles, or utilizing affirmations can all help to foster a loving and upbeat environment. Rituals contribute to the practice's intentional and comprehensive elements.

Yoni mapping makes it possible to have a more customized and deliberate CBD yo-steaming experience while also promoting self-confidence and a deeper understanding of your own body.

CHAPTER 6: ADDRESSING COMMON CONCERNS

When it comes to achieving comprehensive feminine well-being through the use of CBD Yoni Steaming, it is becoming increasingly important to address common difficulties. Managing menstruation discomfort, enhancing libido and sensuality, and achieving hormonal equilibrium with the use of CBD Yoni Steaming are all topics that are covered in this chapter.

Managing Menstrual Discomfort

Menstrual discomfort is a persistent issue for a lot of women. In addition to the possible health advantages of CBD, Yoni Steaming with CBD offers a holistic approach to addressing menstruation discomfort by offering relief through steam. Here's how to deal with this typical worry:

Herbs for Toning and Soothing: Give priority to toning and soothing herbs while blending herbs for CBD Yoni Steaming during menstruation. Calendula, mugwort, chamomile, and rosemary are great options. These plants have analgesic and anti-inflammatory qualities that may help with cramping and pain.

The Inhibitory Effects of CBD: The anti-inflammatory qualities of CBD are well-known, and they can enhance the calming and toning effects of herbal steam. CBD may help lessen the pain and discomfort associated with menstruation by regulating inflammatory responses and interacting with the endocannabinoid system.

Gentle Steaming Techniques: Use kinder techniques while steaming while you are menstruating. Reduce the steam's temperature to make sure you're comfortable and prevent any irritation. Shorter sessions could be advantageous since they enable a calm and gradual experience.

Hydration and Self-Care: To support your body's natural processes during your menstrual cycle, make sure you are drinking plenty of water. To improve general well-being during this time, partake in extra self-care activities like warm baths, light exercise, and mindful pursuits.

Practice Consistency: When using CBD Yoni Steaming to treat menstruation discomfort, consistency is essential. Think about adding the practice to your normal self-care regimen. If you'd like, start with shorter sessions and work your way up to longer ones.

Consultation with Healthcare Providers: See your healthcare practitioner if your menstrual discomfort is severe or ongoing. Although many women find relief with CBD yoni steaming, each person's health situation is unique, and seeking professional advice guarantees a well-rounded approach to well-being.

Improving Libido and Sensuality

Essential components of feminine well-being include a robust feeling of sensuality and libido. You can improve these areas of your self-care routine by including CBD Yoni Steaming. Here's how to handle issues with sensuality and libido:

Stress Reduction and Relaxation: CBD is well-known for its anxiolytic qualities, which support stress reduction and relaxation. When you add CBD to your Yoni Steaming routine, you foster an atmosphere that encourages increased sensuality. Reduced stress is frequently associated with increased libido.

Fragrant Herbs to Enhance the Sensual Experience: To improve the sensory experience, think about incorporating aromatic herbs into your CBD Yoni Steaming blend. In addition to adding to the overall atmosphere, herbs with aromatherapeutic qualities that might enhance mood and sensuality include lavender, rose petals, and jasmine.

Mindful Connection with Your Body: During CBD Yoni Steaming, take part in mindful exercises to help you develop a closer relationship with your body. Breathe deeply, concentrate on the here and now, and accept the practice's comprehensive approach. By improving the mind-body connection, mindfulness contributes to a more positive experience of sensuality.

Open and Intimate Communication: If you're in a relationship, think about having honest and direct conversations about your preferences and aspirations. Examine methods to include CBD yoni steaming in group self-care routines and share your experiences with it.

Self-Examination and Customization: CBD Yoni Steaming offers a chance for introspection and customization. Take this exercise as an opportunity to learn more about what makes you more sensuous and maintains a healthy libido. Try a variety of herbs and CBD doses to see what works best for you.

Consultation with Healthcare Professionals: Seek advice from healthcare professionals if you continue to experience issues with libido or sensuality, particularly if they are hurting your general health. These issues may be caused by hormone imbalances or underlying medical conditions, which can be fully addressed with expert advice.

Balancing Hormones with CBD Yoni Steaming

Hormone balance affects many facets of women's health and is essential for general well-being. When done carefully, CBD yoni steaming may help maintain hormonal balance. Here's how to handle issues with hormone balance:

Understanding the Endocannabinoid System (ECS): The ECS, which is essential for controlling hormone balance, is impacted by interactions between CBD and this system. Numerous physiological functions, such as mood, sleep patterns, and reproductive health, are influenced by the ECS. The ECS is modulated by CBD, which may help maintain hormonal balance.

According to certain studies, CBD has adaptogenic qualities that aid in the body's ability to adjust to stimuli and maintain equilibrium. Hormonal balance can be impacted by stress, and CBD's capacity to lessen stress reactions may tangentially promote hormonal balance.

Selecting Hormone-Balancing Herbs: Take into account herbs that are recognized for their hormone-balancing qualities while blending an herbal mixture for CBD yoni steaming. Certain herbs, such as vitex agnus-castus, red clover, and dong quai, have long been utilized for their beneficial benefits on women's hormonal health.

Personalized Methods: Everybody's hormonal balance is different. With CBD yoni steaming, you may customize the herbal blend to target your unique hormonal issues, allowing for a more individualized approach to healing. Try out various herbs and track your body's reaction over time.

Using CBD-infused Products: External use of CBD-infused oils or salves to the pelvic region may help maintain hormonal balance. Make sure the CBD products you use are of the highest caliber and speak with your medical professionals if you have any particular hormonal issues.

Lifestyle Habits: Take into account lifestyle factors that support hormonal balance in addition to CBD yin steaming. A balanced diet, consistent exercise, enough sleep, and stress reduction are essential for good hormonal health. Yoni steaming with CBD can be a component of a comprehensive approach to wellness.

Professional Advice: Speak with medical professionals or specialists if you have any particular hormonal disorders or concerns. A thorough awareness of your hormonal health is ensured by professional assistance, which also enables customized recommendations.

CHAPTER 7: INTEGRATING CBD YONI STEAMING INTO YOUR SELF-CARE ROUTINE

Using CBD Yoni as an ingredient One of the most effective ways to improve your general well-being and build a deeper connection with your body is to incorporate steaming into your regimen of self-care techniques. This chapter examines the relevance of rituals and ceremonies, as well as the skill of creating a sacred space, developing intentions for your practice, and setting intentions for your practice.

Creating a Sacred Space

Establishing a hallowed area for your CBD A regular practice of yoni steaming is necessary to promote mindfulness and serenity. Here's how to create a place of worship:

Pick a Calm and Quiet Area: Look for a calm and secluded area where you may enjoy CBD yoni steaming without interruptions. By doing this, you can establish a feeling of sanctuary and completely immerse yourself in the practice.

Comfort & Soft Lighting: To create a calming ambiance, use soft, gentle lighting. Think of lighting candles, fairy lights, or low-light bulbs.

To make the space more comfortable, add shawls, blankets, or cushions.

Sensory Elements: Use sensory elements to awaken your senses. Diffuse relaxing essential oils, add fragrant herbs to your CBD Yoni Steaming concoction, or play soothing music or natural noises. The sensory encounter supports mindfulness and relaxation.

Cleanse and Purify the Space: Give the area a quick once-over before your CBD yoni steaming session. Methods like smudging with sage, utilizing essential oils that purify, or using palo santo can accomplish this. A sense of rebirth and sacredness is enhanced by the process of cleaning.

Add Personal Touches: Make your sacred place uniquely yours by adding objects that have special importance for you. These could be symbols that are in line with your aims, crystals, or affirmations. The practice's spiritual and intimate aspects are enhanced by personal objects.

Think About the Seasons and Nature: Align the elements of nature or the seasons with your sacred location. If you're doing CBD Yoni Steaming outside, for instance, take the weather and time of day into account.

Enhancing the practice's grounding and holistic elements is connecting with nature.

Privacy and Limits: Make sure your sacred area is safe and private by drawing distinct boundaries around it. Let people know what you need, and stress to them how important uninterrupted time for self-care is.

Establishing a hallowed area for CBD Yoni steaming enhances the experience's overall advantages by establishing a conscious and intentional habit.

Setting Intentions for Your Practice

Establishing goals for your CBD Yoni Steaming practice gives it more significance and direction. The following is how to make intentions:

Consider Your Objectives: Give some thought to your ultimate objectives and aspirations for implementing CBD yo-yo steaming into your daily self-care regimen. Think about your goals—relaxation, hormonal equilibrium, or a closer relationship with your body.

After you've given your goals some thought, make sure your aims are clear for that particular session. Simple goals like encouraging self-love, relaxation, or taking care of a specific issue like menstruation discomfort might be considered intentions.

Put Your Intentions in Writing: Putting your intentions in writing helps to clarify and increases the intentionality of the exercise. Write down your intentions explicitly in a journal or on paper. Throughout the session, your ideas will be guided by this written statement.

Talk About Your Goals Out Loud: Expressing your goals out loud gives them more weight. Before or during your CBD Yoni Steaming session, declare your intentions out loud. Your vocalization of this action demonstrates your dedication to the discipline.

Emphasis on Positive Affirmations: Include affirmations that are consistent with your goals. Affirmations can improve optimism and a feeling of empowerment. For instance, affirmations such as "I am in sync with my body's natural cycles" can be beneficial if your goal is to support hormonal balance.

Before starting your CBD Yoni Steaming session, focus on yourself by practicing mindful breathing. Intentional and deep breathing helps to settle the mind and fosters the right atmosphere for intention-setting and manifestation.

Reexamine Intentions Following the Session: After the CBD Yoni Steaming session, give your intentions a second thought. Consider if you thought that the experience was in line with your objectives. The relationship between aim setting and the session's overall advantages is strengthened by this reflecting exercise.

By establishing goals for your CBD Yoni Steaming practice, you may fully enjoy the ritual's holistic benefits and give the experience a sense of purpose and mindfulness.

The CBD Yoni Steaming technique is elevated to a spiritual and life-changing event through rituals and ceremonies. Here's how to add ceremonies and rituals to your self-care practice:

- Select Meaningful Dates or Times: If you enjoy CBD yo-y steaming, think about selecting particular dates or times that have symbolic or personal significance for you. This may be connected to moon phases, life milestones, or important events. The ritualistic aspect of the practice is strengthened when it coincides with significant events.

- Establish a Ritualistic Sequence: Come up with a series of actions that revolve around your CBD Yoni Steaming. This could entail clearing the area, making intentions, practicing breathwork, and using particular motions or gestures. The exercise gains depth and structure from a ritualistic process.

- Include Symbolic Aspects: Incorporate symbolic elements that are significant to you personally or culturally. This could involve integrating ritual objects like crystals or sacred fragrances, utilizing particular colors, or inserting symbols that are considered sacred. The practice's ceremonial and spiritual features are enhanced by symbolic elements.

- Sacred Components: Incorporate sacrosanct elements into your ceremonies including the Yoni Steaming of CBD. Acknowledging the elements of earth, water, fire, and air could be one way to do this. Using earthly herbs, steam for water, candle flames for fire, and breath for air are a few examples. This link to the elements gives the ceremony a deeper meaning.

- Express Gratitude: Throughout your CBD Yoni Steaming routines, cultivate an attitude of thankfulness. Give thanks for your body, the environment, and the chance to take care of yourself. Gratitude amplifies the ceremony's good vibe.

- Incorporate Dance or Movement: To establish a physical connection with your body, incorporate dance or movement into your ritual. This might be a dance that goes well with your CBD Yoni Steaming practice, gentle stretching, or sensual motions. Enhancing the mind-body link is movement.

- Post-Ritual Reflection: After your CBD Yoni Steaming ritual is over, give yourself some time to contemplate. Writing in your journal about your feelings, experiences, and realizations helps you incorporate the ritual into your daily self-care practice.

- Exchange Ceremonies with Community Support: You might want to think about sharing your CBD Yoni Steaming rituals with groups that are encouraging. This might include going to women's circles or joining online organizations that appreciate and encourage feminine wellness practices. A sense of community and mutual empowerment is fostered by shared rites.

Your CBD Yoni Steaming practice can be elevated above a simple self-care regimen by incorporating rituals and ceremonies, which embrace the transforming and spiritual components of feminine well-being.

CHAPTER 8: BEYOND PERSONAL WELLNESS - COMMUNITY AND CONNECTION

When it comes to the investigation of CBD Yoni Steaming, the journey goes beyond the sphere of personal well-being and into the realms of community and connection. Within the context of CBD Yoni Steaming, this chapter digs at the transforming impact of sharing experiences, the significance of constructing a supportive community, and the role that education plays in empowering others.

The Power of Sharing Experiences

The ability of CBD Yoni Steaming to alter frequently goes beyond personal experiences, having a beneficial knock-on effect that can benefit others. By talking about your experiences with CBD yoni steaming, you can break taboos, connect with others, and inspire them to take charge of their wellness journeys. How to do it is as follows:

- Breaking Taboos and Stigmas: Like many holistic therapies, CBD yoni steaming may be shrouded in taboos or stigmas. You help to dismantle these barriers by freely sharing your experiences. Sincere talks contribute to the normalization of the discourse surrounding feminine well-being and self-care.

- Motivating Others to Investigate Wellness: People who are apprehensive or inquisitive about exploring holistic wellness techniques can find motivation in their own experience with CBD Yoni Steaming. By sharing how your journey has improved your life, you can inspire others to take similar steps.

- Establishing a Safe Space for Conversation: Honest Talk about CBD Yoni Steaming establishes a conversation-safe environment. Promote inquiry, inquisitiveness, and a range of viewpoints. Without fear of rejection, people can open up about their ideas, worries, and experiences in a friendly setting.

- Empathy and Connection: In communities, sharing your experiences promotes empathy and a sense of belonging. Others may identify with your struggles, victories, and revelations, forging a common understanding of the complex concept of feminine well-being.

- Emphasizing Diversity of Experiences: Each person's CBD Yoni Steaming experience is distinct. You advance a more comprehensive grasp of the practice by sharing a variety of narratives. Because of this variety, people can investigate the subtleties of CBD yoni steaming and choose methods that work for them.

- Online Communities and Platforms: To share your experiences, use social media, online communities, or online platforms. These platforms offer a global forum where people may interact, exchange ideas, and gain knowledge from each other's experiences.

- Encouraging Body Positivity: CBD Conversations Yoni steaming has the potential to advance body positivity. Stress the value of self-care routines that promote a healthy relationship with one's own body and the celebration of the female form.

Building a Supportive Community

establishing a welcoming neighborhood around CBD Yoni Steaming fosters a feeling of empowerment and mutual understanding among participants. Here's how to cultivate a community that is encouraging:

- Creating Safe Venues: Create safe spaces for conversations on CBD yoni steaming, whether they take place online or in person. Promote candid dialogue, attentive hearing, and the exchange of differing viewpoints. People can express themselves in safe settings without worrying about being judged.

- Encouraging Peer Support: In a community, peer support is really helpful. Invite people to talk about their struggles, inquiries, and victories. Peer support helps people in the community learn from one another and builds a sense of togetherness.

- Putting Together Workshops and Events: Plan CBD Yoni Steaming-related workshops or events. These events give locals a chance to interact face-to-face, exchange stories, and pick the brains of subject matter experts. Workshop subjects may include CBD integration, mindfulness techniques, and herbal mixtures.

- Working Together with Wellness Practitioners: To offer the community insightful information, and collaborate with herbalists, holistic health specialists, or wellness practitioners. The community can benefit from the varied viewpoints and increased understanding of guest speakers or facilitators on feminine wellness.

- Developing Digital Materials: To spread knowledge about CBD Yoni Steaming, provide digital resources including webinars, articles, and tutorials. Accessible resources serve as a point of reference for further conversations and aid in the education of community members.

- Creating Community Guidelines: Clearly state the values that encourage tolerance, acceptance, and a judgment-free environment. Community members are supported and encouraged to express themselves authentically when guidelines are followed.

- Promoting Collaboration: Promote cooperation among community members. This could be cooperative efforts to advance the general well-being of community members, shared experiences, or group projects.

- Honoring Milestones: Within the community, honor both individual and group accomplishments. Acknowledge successes, personal development, and the beneficial effects of CBD Yoni Steaming on community members' well-being.

Educating Others on CBD Yoni Steaming

Demystifying CBD Yoni Steaming and enabling people to make knowledgeable decisions about their health depend heavily on education. Here's how you can help spread knowledge among others:

Information Exchange Act responsibly: Give accuracy and accountability a priority when disseminating information on CBD Yoni Steaming. Make sure the data you provide is derived from reliable sources, original research, and firsthand knowledge. Conscientious sharing fosters trust among neighbors.

Organizing Educational Events: Conduct educational events in your neighborhood to learn more about the background, advantages, and science of CBD Yoni Steaming. To improve understanding, these seminars may have interactive discussions, Q&A periods, and special guests.

Working with Experts: Assist those who are knowledgeable in CBD, herbalism, and holistic wellness. Professionals can answer inquiries, offer insightful commentary, and provide a sophisticated grasp of CBD yoni steaming. Their experience gives educational programs more legitimacy.

Producing Educational Content: Write educational articles, infographics, or movies that can be shared across a range of media. Pay attention to answering frequently asked concerns, dispelling misconceptions, and offering helpful advice to people who are considering CBD yo-steaming.

Providing Beginner Workshops: Create workshops, especially for those who are just learning about the idea of CBD Yoni Steaming. Address fundamental subjects, safety measures, and useful advice to establish a friendly entrance point for individuals who are ready to learn.

Using Social Media for Education: Spread instructional materials by utilizing social media platforms. Visually captivating and easily shared content can be found on platforms like YouTube, Instagram, and TikTok, reaching a large audience.

Having Open Discussions: Encourage discussions about CBD Yoni Steaming both inside and outside of your community. Urge others to participate in the continuing discussion, voice their concerns, and ask questions. Open discussions encourage a culture of lifelong learning.

Taking Care of Misconceptions: Be proactive in taking care of any misunderstandings or false information that may exist regarding CBD Yoni Steaming. Dispelling myths and ensuring that people have accurate information to make educated decisions are two benefits of open and honest communication.

Encouraging Inclusivity: Take an inclusive stance when it comes to education, acknowledging that people can have different experiences, backgrounds, and worldviews. Establish a welcoming atmosphere for all, and design instructional materials to appeal to a wide range of learners.

You add to the larger story of CBD Yoni Steaming by actively engaging in community-building, experience-sharing, and teaching. This promotes a culture of empowerment, understanding, and connection.

CHAPTER 9: FAQS AND TROUBLESHOOTING

There is a possibility that consumers will have questions and concerns when they begin their experience with CBD Yoni Steaming. The purpose of this chapter is to provide troubleshooting help and answers to frequently asked issues to ensure a smooth and pleasurable experience.

Common Questions about CBD Yoni Steaming

Q1: *What is CBD Yoni Steaming, and how does it work?*

A1: CBD Yoni steaming, also called vaginal steaming, is a holistic self-care technique where you sit over a bowl of steaming water that has been infused with different herbs and CBD. It is said that the warm steam enhances general feminine well-being, supports menstruation health, and encourages relaxation. Hemp-based CBD is added because of its possible relaxing and anti-inflammatory effects.

Q2: *Is CBD Yoni Steaming safe?*

A2: CBD Yoni Steaming is usually believed to be safe for a large number of people when it is performed thoughtfully and with attention to safety requirements. The selection of CBD products of high quality, the utilization of suitable herbs, and the adherence to the prescribed criteria for temperature and time are all quite significant. However, before introducing CBD Yoni Steaming into their routine, persons who have particular health conditions or concerns should be sure to check with their healthcare experts.

Q3: *How often should I practice CBD Yoni Steaming?*

A3: Following one's preferences and requirements, the frequency of CBD Yoni Steaming should be determined. Weekly sessions may be beneficial for some people, while others could find that monthly sessions are sufficient for them. Pay attention to the signals that your body sends you, and alter the frequency accordingly. Avoid steaming for an extended period because it can irritate.

Q4: *Can CBD Yoni Steaming be done during menstruation?*

A4: Yes, it is possible to do CBD Yoni Steaming while you are menstruating; however, it is vital to alter the practice such that it allows you to feel comfortable. When you want to assist relaxation, use herbs that are toning and relaxing, and think about using a softer steam temperature. Personal preferences can vary, therefore it is important to pay attention to your body and select the option that seems most appropriate for you at this particular moment.

Q5: *Can I use any type of CBD product for Yoni Steaming?*

A5: When using Yoni Steaming, it is advisable to utilize CBD products that are of high quality and pure. The CBD product you purchase mustn't contain any chemicals, toxins, or synthetic components. There is a preference for oils that contain CBD or herbal mixes that have been specifically produced for Yoni Steaming because these products are formulated to be both safe and effective.

Q6: *What are some potential benefits of CBD Yoni Steaming?*

A6: The practice of CBD Yoni Steaming has been linked to several potential advantages, including the promotion of a sense of overall well-being, relaxation, and support for menstrual cycles. It is possible that the anti-inflammatory qualities of CBD could help alleviate discomfort, and the ritualistic aspect of steaming can make self-care routines more effective.

Q7: *Can CBD Yoni Steaming help with fertility?*

A7: Even though CBD Yoni Steaming is not a treatment that is guaranteed to increase fertility, some people choose to add it to their fertility journey as a holistic practice. It is possible that the steaming session, which is known for its calming effects, will provide emotional support. Additionally, the herbal blend may contain some herbs that are historically connected with fertility.

Q8: *Can I create my herbal blends for CBD Yoni Steaming?*

A8: Yes, you can make your herbal mixtures using CBD Yoni Steaming. Be sure to select herbs that are well-known for their safety and the possible benefits they may offer. You should take into consideration your goals, your tastes, and any particular issues that you might have. By conducting studies and consulting with herbalists, you can build a blend that is specifically suited to your requirements.

Addressing Challenges and Concerns

- **Challenge 1:** Pain or Angst During or Following Steaming

- **Possible Causes:** The steam temperature may be too high, or the herbal blend may be too strong.

- **Troubleshooting:** Shorten the period or lower the steam temperature. Add more calming herbs to the herbal blend, such as calendula or chamomile.

- **Challenge 2:** Lack of Desired Effects

- **Possible Causes:** People react differently, and it could take some time to see the desired results.

- **Troubleshooting:** Try out various CBD concentrations, herbal mixes, and session lengths. After some time, practice regularly and evaluate the effect on your well-being again.

- **Challenge 3:** Uncertainty about Herb Choices

- **Possible Causes:** Due to ignorance, selecting herbs for Yoni Steaming might be quite difficult.

- **Troubleshooting:** Speak with herbalists, do your homework from reliable sources, or take a look at prepackaged herbal mixtures made specifically for yoni steaming. Commence with popular herbs such as chamomile, lavender, or rosemary.

- **Challenge 4:** Difficulty in Creating a Ritualistic Atmosphere

- **Possible Causes:** Establishing a sacred area could seem difficult or strange.

- **Troubleshooting:** Begin modestly by adding components such as aromatherapy, soothing music, or soft lighting. As you get more at ease with the ceremonial part, gradually go into greater detail with these components.

- **Challenge 5:** Concerns about Privacy or Judgment

- **Possible Causes:** Fear of being judged or uneasy about the behavior in public areas.

- **Troubleshooting:** Select a safe, quiet area for your practice. Share your needs with people who are close to you and stress the value of having undisturbed time for self-care.

- **Challenge 6:** Sensitivity to CBD or Herbs

- **Possible Causes:** Individual sensitivities or allergies to certain herbs or CBD.

- **Troubleshooting:** Before utilizing new plants or CBD products, do patch tests. Lower the concentrations at first and see how your body reacts. Speak with medical professionals if the sensitivity continues.

- **Challenge 7:** Difficulty in Maintaining Consistency

- **Possible Causes:** Busy schedules or a lack of established routines.

- **Troubleshooting:** Schedule your CBD Yoni Steaming sessions at certain times, include them in your current self-care regimens, and let people know when you need help. Intentional preparation is frequently the first step in developing consistency.

Due to the diversity of individual experiences and interests, difficulties must be approached with a personalized strategy. You may maximize the advantages of CBD Yoni Steaming while promoting a positive and powerful experience by troubleshooting and customizing the practice to suit your needs.

CONCLUSION

As we get to the end of our thorough investigation into CBD Yoni Steaming, we find ourselves at the nexus of traditional knowledge and contemporary self-care. This ground-breaking exploration of feminine wellness has revealed a practice that goes beyond the physical, enabling people to set out on a comprehensive path of self-actualization and empowerment.

Summary of the Main Ideas:

We started our adventure by learning the fundamentals of Yoni Steaming, an age-old technique that benefits women's physical, emotional, and spiritual well-being. We investigated the incorporation of CBD, a non-psychoactive substance with possible soothing and anti-inflammatory effects, taking the practice to new heights. As the potential advantages of CBD yoni steaming became apparent, they included enhanced sensuality, better sleep, assistance for menstruation, and a healthy mind-body connection.

The fundamentals of Yoni Steaming have revealed an old ritual that links us to a variety of cultural traditions and offers historical background and an understanding of its workings. We investigated the medicinal qualities of CBD, learning about its relationship to the endocannabinoid system and its possible advantages for the well-being of women. Helpful advice for beginning a CBD regimen From necessary equipment to selecting the best CBD products, Yoni Steaming gave people the knowledge they needed to engage in a safe and successful activity.

Creating unique DIY CBD Yoni Steaming recipes has become a craft, enabling customization according to personal tastes and requirements. We investigated the deep relationship we have with our bodies by learning about body language, menstrual cycle awareness, and Yoni mapping. Managing common issues including libido enhancement, menstrual discomfort management, and hormone balance demonstrated the comprehensive approach of CBD Yoni Steaming.

By establishing a sacred place, making intentions, and participating in rituals and ceremonies, integration into self-care routines turned the practice into an intentional and conscious one. We explored the transforming potential of sharing experiences, creating supportive networks, and educating others in addition to personal healing. For individuals who were unfamiliar with CBD Yoni Steaming, FAQs and troubleshooting offered answers to frequently asked queries and issues, guaranteeing a comforting and happy experience.

To sum up, CBD Yoni Steaming is a call to recognize and enjoy the complex fabric of feminine wellness, not just a discipline. Each steaming session brings forth a sense of empowerment, self-love, and holistic well-being as it is an investigation of the mind, body, and soul. May this book be your traveling companion, providing direction, motivation, and a solid base for accepting the life-changing experience that is yet to come. Through the age-old practice of CBD yoni steaming, may people who set out on this journey discover empowerment, a sense of connection, and a revitalized sense of well-being.